MR. MEN™ LITTLE MISS™ © THOIP (a SANRIO company)

Little Miss Mum-to-Be © 2021 THOIP (a SANRIO company)
Printed and published under license from Penguin Random House LLC
Published in Great Britain by Farshore
An imprint of HarperCollins*Publishers*
1 London Bridge Street, London SE1 9GF
www.farshore.co.uk

HarperCollins*Publishers*
1st Floor, Watermarque Building, Ringsend Road
Dublin 4, Ireland

ISBN 978 1 4052 9967 1
Printed in Italy
002

LITTLE MISS
MUM-TO-BE

Roger Hargreaves

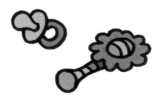

Original concept and illustrations by
Roger Hargreaves

Written by
Sarah Daykin and Lizzie Daykin

Spring was springing, buds were blooming and lambs were leaping in Sprogland.

Mother Hen was paying a visit to the Little Misses.

'Cluck, cluck, cluck,' she went, clucking her way around the village, sprinkling her magical seed.

She had blessed the Little Misses with the miracle of new life, and they couldn't wait to meet their little bundles of joy.

If only Mother Hen had prepared them for the constipation, sleep deprivation and insatiable cravings for beige foods.

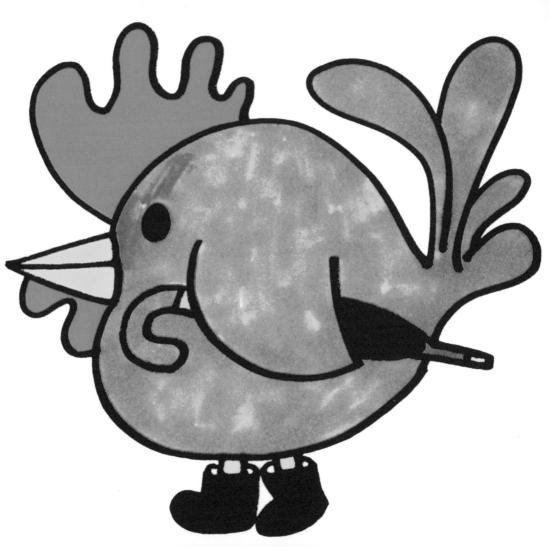

Little Miss Wise was overwhelmed with happiness at the news of her pregnancy.

She was a little concerned that she had no idea what she was doing, her social life was over and her career would go down the plughole ... but other than that she was taking it in her stride.

She was strolling back from her 12 week scan (after being sick in a nearby bush), thinking about the little pink blob she'd seen growing inside of her.

'I wonder what I'll call my baby?' she thought. 'Maybe I should call it Brie ... and it'll grow up to be a famous cheesemonger!'

'BLEURGH!' retched Little Miss Wise. 'Maybe I should stop thinking about cheese.'

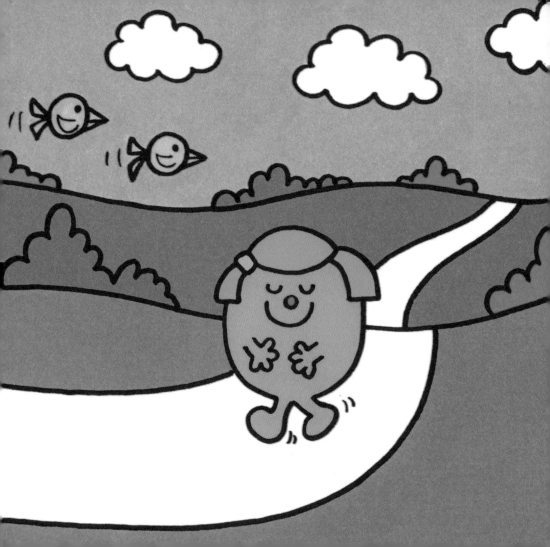

Little Miss Curious wanted to know what to expect when expecting and decided to ask Dr Google.

Six hours later she'd signed up to Mumsgas, Babybabble and Smothercare, feeling more confused than when she'd started.

Ping! Another notification comparing her baby to the size of a kumquat.

Should she buy the £8000 pushchair with six-wheel drive? Or should she spend the money on a gender reveal party with exploding glitter bombs and a live orchestra?

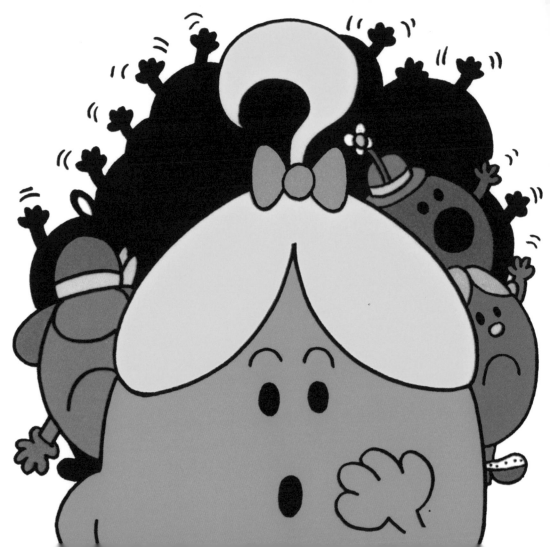

Little Miss Star took a snap of her bump in the mirror for her photo diary. She felt like she was expanding faster than the big bang and wondered if she'd soon be visible from space.

Her hormones were all over the place and she couldn't stop sweating, but her partner insisted she was glowing.

'It's alright for them to say,' thought Little Miss Star. 'They're not the one with a baby using their bladder as a punch bag.'

Just then her partner came in with a cup of tea and offered to give her a foot massage.

Maybe being pregnant wasn't so bad after all.

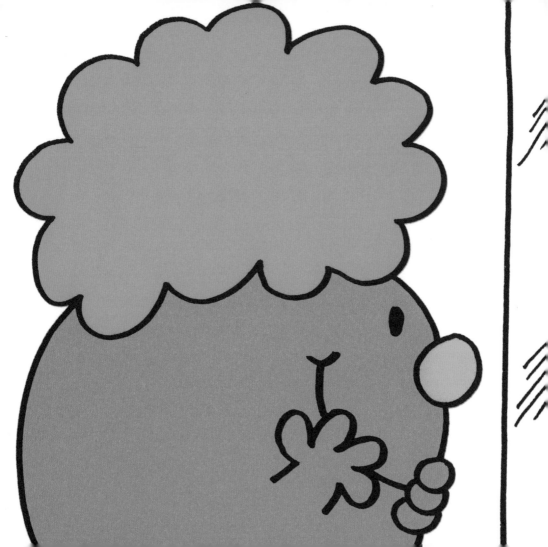

Little Miss Stubborn had a craving and she would not rest until it was satisfied. Her stomach led her to Mr Strong's house, who always had a well-stocked fridge.

He made exactly what she asked for: a big plate of eggs (338 to be precise), with a side of chocolate-covered chicken livers, topped with whipped cream and a sprinkling of dirt.

'Deeeelicious!' said Little Miss Stubborn, happily shovelling it into her mouth.

'Can I get you anything else?' asked Mr Strong, nervously.

'Yes, same again please!'

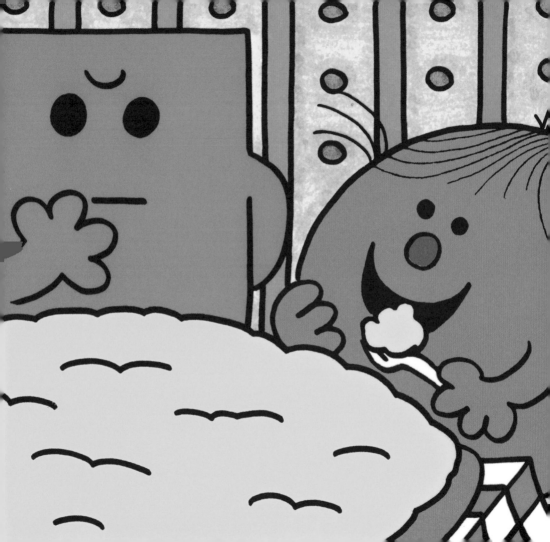

Little Miss Tidy was planning the perfect stress-free birth and started every morning with detox yoga.

'I love this class. Great excuse for a nap isn't it?' said Little Miss Chatterbox, who was pregnant with her fifth child.

'I wish!' said Little Miss Tidy, clutching her pregnancy bible. 'After this I've got to rehearse my birth plan, do my positive affirmations and practise hypno-breathing!'

'Or I could treat you to a slice of cake,' said Little Miss Chatterbox, breezily. 'I'll tell you about the time I sneezed and gave birth to my twins in a car park.'

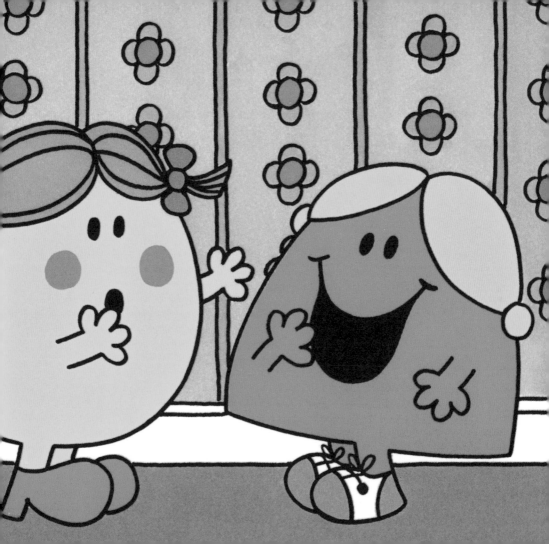

Mr Brave hesitated nervously outside the door of his first antenatal class.

'Come on in,' said the class leader. 'We're just about to cover perineal massage.'

He sat down next to Mr Greedy who was asking questions and taking notes. 'Is it true you can eat the afterbirth?'

Mr Brave stared at his shoes (even though he didn't have any) and Mr Muddle turned a deeper shade of green.

Then the leader handed Mr Brave a plastic baby. 'Make sure you support its neck,' she said.

Boing, boing, boing! He watched in horror as its head detached and bounced across the floor. This was going to be harder than he'd thought.

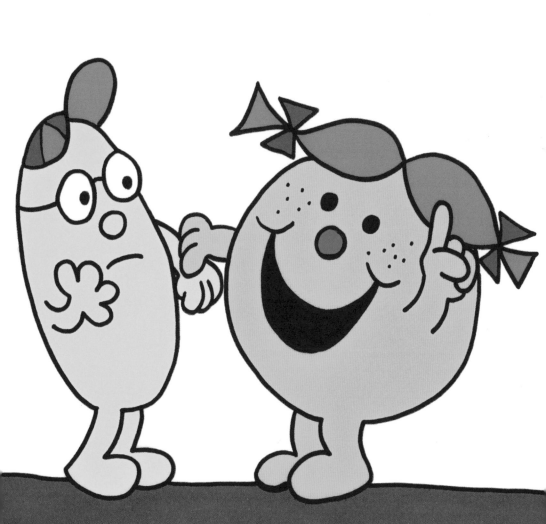

Little Miss Curious was as overdue as her Blockbuster video, her Windows 95 library book and her team winning the World Cup.

She had eaten a vat of pineapple vindaloo, drunk a gallon of raspberry leaf tea and even walked up her stairs like a crab, but there was still no sign of the baby.

She was now quite literally the size of a house.

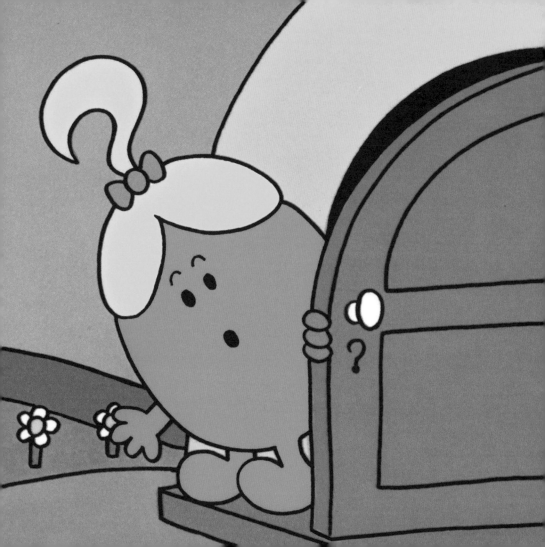

Little Miss Greedy had been having contractions for six hours when she suddenly felt her waters break.

'I think I need to go to hospital!' she said, starting to panic.

'Not to worry my love,' said Mr Greedy, blowing up a birthing ball. 'I know exactly what to do. I'll just put on some relaxing whale song.'

'I don't want to listen to any bloody whale song, I want to go to hospital!'

'Ah yes,' said Mr Greedy. 'I was warned you might get a bit upset, but I won't take it personally.'

'Good ... THEN GET ME TO THE %&*$@$* HOSPITAL!!!'

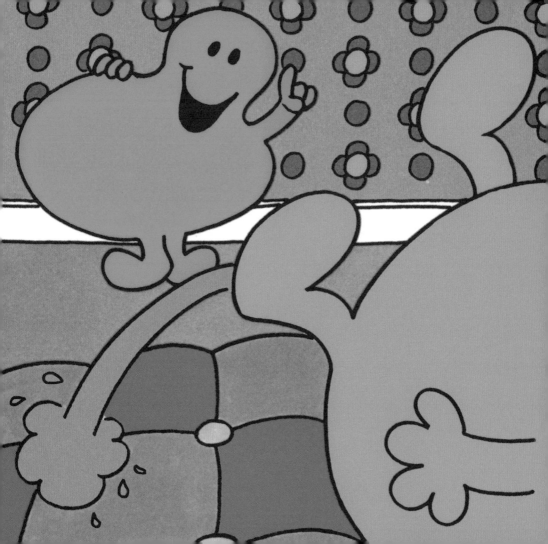

Thankfully Little Miss Greedy did get to the %&*$@$* hospital and was in the capable hands of the midwives.

She had now turned feral, ripping off all of her clothes and panting like a wild animal.

'You're doing really well,' said Dr Cool, calmly.

Mr Greedy had hurriedly set up his video camera at what he was now referring to as 'the business end' and was pleased to have secured a front row seat.

Luckily he pressed record just before he passed out.

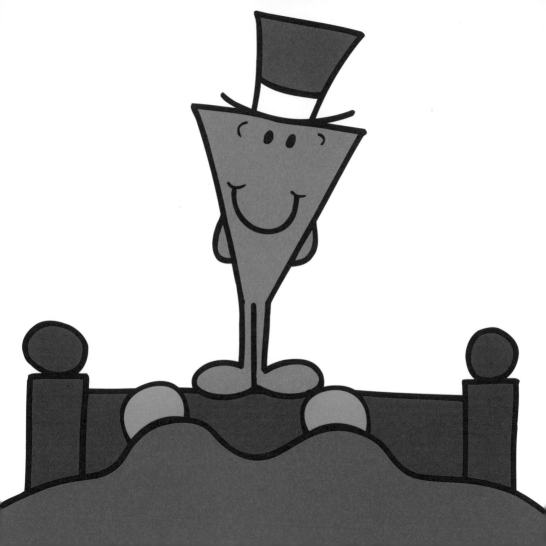

When Mr Greedy finally came round, he was handed the most beautiful thing he'd ever seen ... a plate of buttery marmalade toast. And then he was handed his newborn baby.

'Look at its chubby little fingers,' he said, his heart melting. 'They look just like mine.'

He couldn't stop telling everyone how proud he was of his wife.

'She was incredible from start to finish, totally unflappable, cool as a cucumber!'

It was only once the Greedys got home that they realised the enormity of the task ahead of them ... starting with their first nappy.

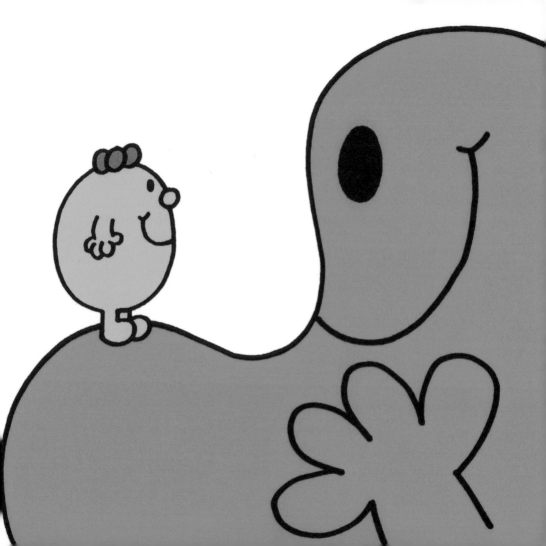

It was a momentous day for Little Miss Quick, who'd managed to brush her teeth, go to the loo and put a bow in her hair at record speed, all before the baby needed feeding again.

She was starting to feel a bit like a pair of boobs on legs and had developed a newfound respect for cows.

At least she could have some adult conversation with her Mum friends, even if it was only about nappy rash and poo explosions.

And she was grateful for the production line of homemade lasagne her friends and family kept delivering.

Maybe tomorrow she'd attempt the insurmountable challenge of changing out of her pyjamas.

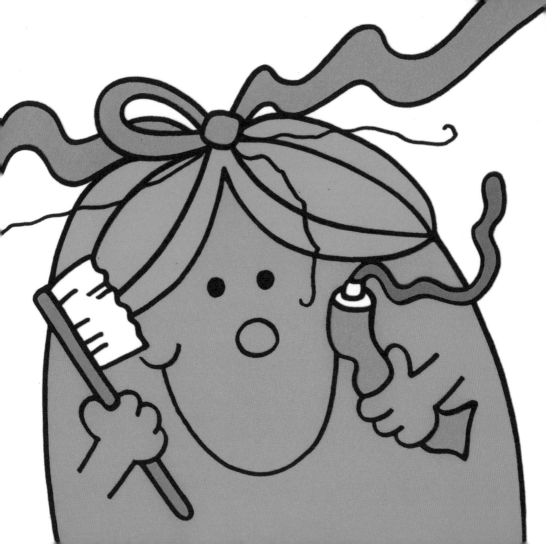

Mr Small and Mr Tickle were comparing notes on the challenges of being a new dad.

'I've had 20 minutes sleep in 3 days,' said Mr Small.

'Lucky you, my baby is so full of wind I spend every night squeezing it like a bagpipe,' said Mr Tickle.

'Tell me about it. How can so much poo come out of something so small?!'

'Yesterday, I went to baby sensory class and paid £10 for the privilege of wafting a ribbon in my baby's face.'

'Eurgh! There's nothing worse than being around other people's children ... but my baby's great though.'

'Yep mine too, wouldn't change it for the world.'

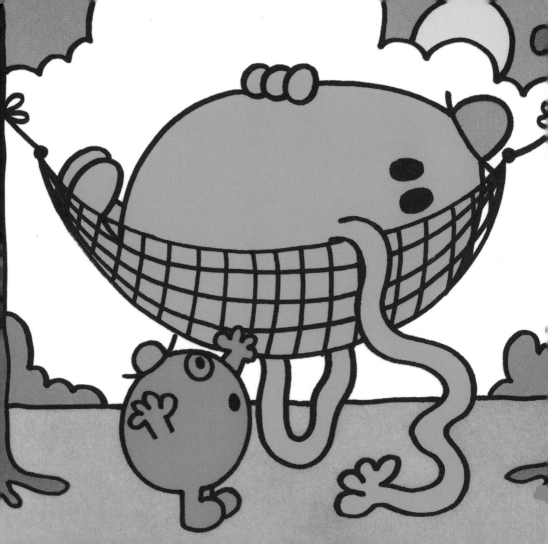

The grandparents couldn't wait to meet their granddaughter and share their unsolicited parental advice.

Grandma, who was insisting on being called 'Fab-ma', was already asking why the baby wasn't wearing the knitted jumper she'd sent.

'She'll catch a cold!' she said handing the baby to 'Great-pa'.

'Look at that honker,' he said. 'She's the spit of Uncle Ugly.'

'It's like being a new parent all over again,' said Fab-ma finishing her fiftieth cup of tea and helping herself to another biscuit.

'Exhausting isn't it!' said Great-pa. 'Anyway, looks like her nappy needs changing, so we'd better be off.'

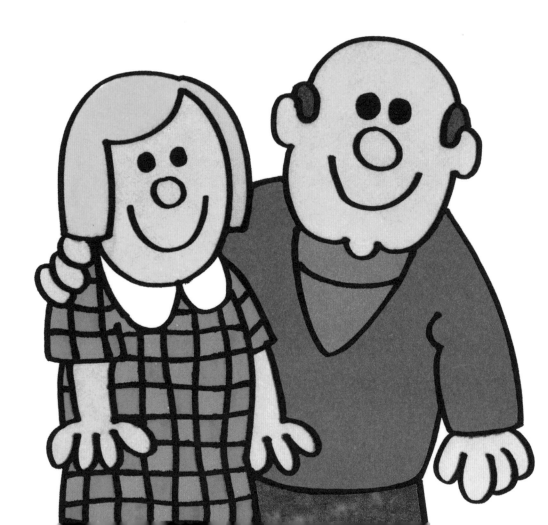

Little Miss Tidy hadn't planned on having a nocturnal baby. In fact there were quite a few things that hadn't gone to plan ...

She certainly hadn't prepared to go into labour in a cake shop, or for Little Miss Chatterbox to hijack a bus to get her to hospital. She'd even ditched her drug-free birth for a drug-free-for-all birth.

But she also hadn't anticipated the heart-exploding love she would feel for her baby. Or how useful her yoga mat would be for changing nappies.

One thing was for sure, having a baby was hard and she'd never be doing it again …

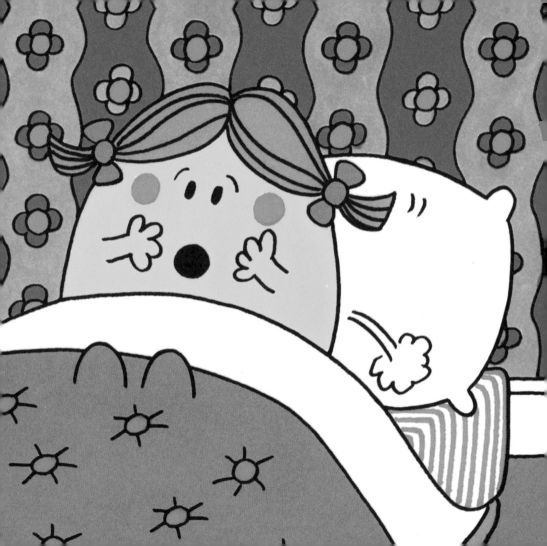

... Until the next one.

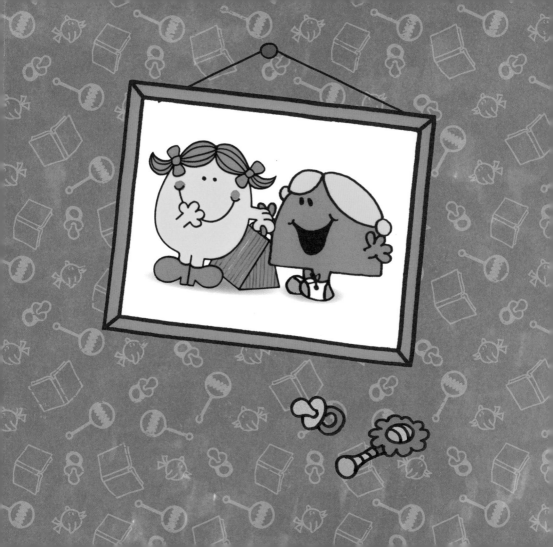

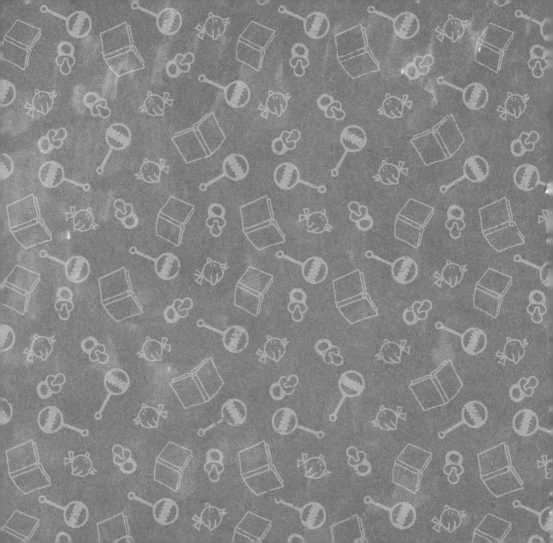